30 MINUTE GESTATIONAL DIABETES COOKBOOK

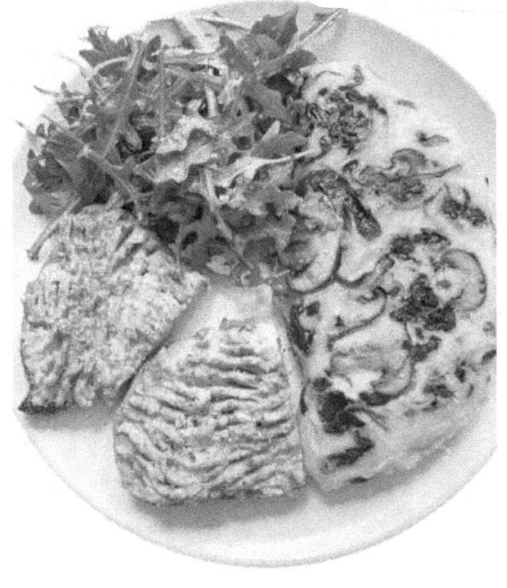

Wholesome 30-Minute Gestational Diabetes-Friendly Meals

Linda Carlucci

Copyright © 2024 by Linda Carlucci

DISCLAIMER

This cookbook is intended to provide general information and recipes.

The recipes provided in this cookbook are not intended to replace or be a substitute for medical advice from a physician.

The reader should consult a healthcare professional for any specific medical advice, diagnosis or treatment.

Any specific dietary advice provided in this cookbook is not intended to replace or be a substitute for medical advice from a physician.

The author is not responsible or liable for any adverse effects experienced by readers of this cookbook as a result of following the recipes or dietary advice provided.

The author makes no representations or warranties of any kind (express or implied) as to the accuracy, completeness, reliability or suitability of the recipes provided in this cookbook.

The author disclaims any and all liability for any damages arising out of the use or misuse of the recipes provided in this cookbook. The reader must also take care to ensure that the recipes provided in this cookbook are prepared and cooked safely.

The recipes provided in this cookbook are for informational purposes only and should not be used as a substitute for professional medical advice, diagnosis or treatment.

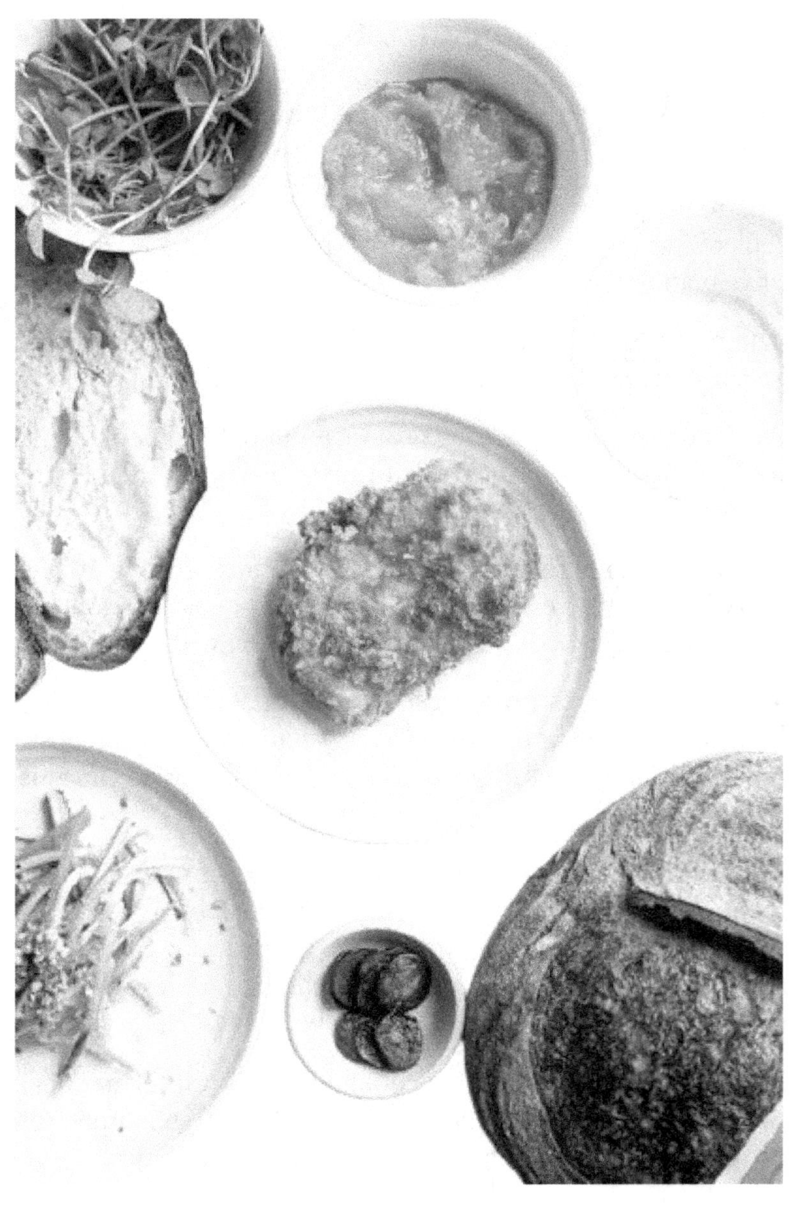

TABLE OF CONTENTS

INTRODUCTION

Gestational diabetes, a condition emerging during pregnancy, poses a significant health concern for both mothers and infants.

This metabolic disorder is characterized by elevated blood sugar levels that if left unmanaged, can lead to various complications.

Understanding the intricacies of gestational diabetes is paramount in mitigating its adverse effects on maternal and fetal health.

During pregnancy, the body undergoes profound physiological changes, affecting insulin sensitivity.

Gestational diabetes arises when the pancreas fails to produce sufficient insulin to regulate the increased glucose levels.

This condition not only jeopardizes the well-being of the mother but also exposes the developing fetus to a myriad of potential complications.

The negative impact of gestational diabetes extends beyond the immediate health risks. Women diagnosed with this condition are at an elevated risk of developing type 2 diabetes later in life, emphasizing the long-term implications.

Moreover, infants born to mothers with gestational diabetes may face immediate health challenges, such as macrosomia (excessive birth weight), respiratory distress syndrome, and hypoglycemia.

The repercussions of gestational diabetes extend to the realm of public health, as the prevalence of this condition is on the rise globally.

Finally, factors such as obesity, sedentary lifestyles, and genetic predispositions contribute to its increasing incidence.

Consequently, there is a pressing need for heightened awareness, effective screening, and comprehensive management strategies to curb the escalating impact of gestational diabetes on maternal and neonatal health.

CHAPTER 1

RISKS ASSOCIATED WITH GESTATIONAL DIABETES

1. **Macrosomia (Large Birth Weight):** Gestational diabetes can lead to macrosomia, where the baby grows excessively large, increasing the risk of birth complications for both mother and child.

2. **Hypoglycemia in Newborns:** Babies born to mothers with gestational diabetes may experience low blood sugar levels (hypoglycemia) shortly after birth, requiring careful monitoring and intervention.

3. **Preterm Birth:** Gestational diabetes is linked to an increased risk of preterm labor and delivery, potentially impacting the baby's development and health.

4. **Respiratory Distress Syndrome:** Infants born to mothers with gestational diabetes have a higher likelihood of experiencing respiratory distress syndrome, a condition affecting the baby's ability to breathe properly.

5. **Type 2 Diabetes Risk for Mothers:** Women with gestational diabetes are at an elevated risk of developing type 2 diabetes later in life, underscoring the importance of long-term health management.

6. **Preeclampsia:** There is an increased risk of developing preeclampsia, a serious condition characterized by high blood pressure and potential organ damage, during pregnancy.

7. **Polyhydramnios:** Gestational diabetes can contribute to polyhydramnios, an excess of amniotic fluid, increasing the risk of complications during delivery.

8. **Neonatal Hypocalcemia:** Babies born to mothers with gestational diabetes may face an increased risk of neonatal hypocalcemia, affecting calcium levels in the blood.

9. **Childhood Obesity:** Children born to mothers with gestational diabetes may have a higher susceptibility to obesity and metabolic issues in childhood and beyond.

10. **Gestational Hypertension:** Gestational diabetes is associated with an elevated risk of developing

gestational hypertension, which can have implications for both maternal and fetal health.

11. **Long-Term Cardiovascular Risks for Mothers:** Women with a history of gestational diabetes have an increased likelihood of developing cardiovascular issues later in life.

12. **Increased Risk of Stillbirth:** Untreated or poorly managed gestational diabetes may elevate the risk of stillbirth, emphasizing the importance of vigilant medical care.

13. **Birth Trauma:** The risk of birth injuries, such as shoulder dystocia, is higher in pregnancies complicated by gestational diabetes, necessitating careful monitoring and potentially intervention during delivery.

14. **Childhood Diabetes:** Offspring born to mothers with gestational diabetes have a higher risk of developing type 2 diabetes in childhood or adolescence.

15. **Maternal Mental Health:** The stress associated with managing gestational diabetes, coupled with

concerns about the baby's health, may contribute to maternal anxiety and stress during pregnancy.

WHAT IS INSULIN RESISTANCE

Insulin resistance is a metabolic condition in which cells throughout the body exhibit a reduced response to insulin, a hormone crucial for regulating blood sugar levels.

In a healthy metabolic process, insulin facilitates the uptake of glucose from the bloodstream into cells, allowing them to use it for energy. However, in insulin resistance, this mechanism becomes less effective, leading to elevated blood sugar levels and potential health complications.

Several factors contribute to insulin resistance, including genetic predisposition, obesity, sedentary lifestyle, and certain medical conditions.

As adipose tissue increases, it releases substances that can interfere with insulin's action. Additionally, physical inactivity and a diet high in refined carbohydrates and sugars can exacerbate insulin resistance.

The consequences of insulin resistance extend beyond impaired glucose regulation. The body compensates by producing more insulin to overcome the reduced effectiveness, leading to elevated insulin levels in the bloodstream. This hyperinsulinemia is associated with various health risks, including increased inflammation, high blood pressure, and abnormal lipid profiles.

Again, insulin resistance is a central feature of type 2 diabetes, as prolonged resistance can eventually lead to inadequate insulin production by the pancreas.

Moreover, it plays a role in the development of metabolic syndrome, a cluster of conditions that heighten the risk of heart disease, stroke, and type 2 diabetes.

Detecting insulin resistance typically involves assessing blood glucose and insulin levels. Lifestyle modifications, such as adopting a balanced diet, engaging in regular physical activity, and maintaining a healthy weight, are fundamental in managing insulin resistance.

In some cases, medications may be prescribed to enhance insulin sensitivity or regulate blood sugar levels.

Understanding and addressing insulin resistance is crucial for preventing and managing various metabolic disorders. By promoting lifestyle changes and early intervention, you can mitigate the associated health risks and improve overall metabolic health.

THE IMPACT OF FOOD ON YOUR BLOOD SUGAR

1. **Carbohydrate Content:** Foods rich in carbohydrates have a significant impact on blood sugar levels. Carbohydrates are broken down into glucose during digestion, causing a rapid increase in blood sugar.

2. **Glycemic Index (GI):** The glycemic index gauges the speed at which a food containing carbohydrates increases blood sugar levels. High-GI foods lead to a swift spike in blood glucose, while low-GI foods cause a slower, more gradual increase.

3. **Fiber Content:** Foods high in fiber, such as whole grains, fruits, and vegetables, can help stabilize blood sugar levels by slowing down the absorption of glucose.

4. **Protein Intake:** Including protein in meals can help moderate blood sugar levels. Protein slows the

digestion of carbohydrates, preventing a rapid surge in glucose.

5. **Fat Content:** Foods rich in fat can delay the absorption of sugar, leading to a more gradual increase in blood glucose. However, excessive fat intake may contribute to insulin resistance over time.

6. **Meal Composition:** Balanced meals that combine carbohydrates, proteins, and fats in appropriate proportions can help regulate blood sugar levels more effectively than meals that are skewed toward one macronutrient.

7. **Portion Size:** Overeating, even with healthy foods, can lead to an excess intake of carbohydrates, causing elevated blood sugar levels.

8. **Meal Timing:** Spreading food intake throughout the day and avoiding prolonged periods without eating can help maintain stable blood sugar levels.

9. **Food Processing:** Highly processed foods, especially those containing refined sugars and flours, can cause rapid spikes in blood sugar due to their quick digestion and absorption.

10. **Artificial Sweeteners:** While non-nutritive sweeteners don't directly affect blood sugar, they may influence insulin response and cravings, potentially impacting overall dietary choices.

11. **Alcohol Consumption:** Moderate alcohol intake can affect blood sugar levels, causing fluctuations that may require careful monitoring, especially for individuals with diabetes.

12. **Caffeine:** Some studies suggest that caffeine may impact insulin sensitivity, potentially affecting blood sugar levels. However, individual responses can vary.

13. **Hydration:** Staying well-hydrated is essential for overall health and can indirectly influence blood sugar regulation. Dehydration may lead to elevated glucose levels.

14. **Nutrient Density:** Choosing nutrient-dense foods provides essential vitamins and minerals that support overall health and may contribute to better blood sugar control.

15. **Individual Response:** Each person's body responds differently to foods. Monitoring blood sugar levels

and paying attention to how specific foods affect you personally is crucial for managing blood sugar effectively.

FOODS THAT SPIKE YOUR BLOOD SUGAR LEVEL TO AVOID

1. **Sugary Beverages:** Sodas, fruit juices, and sweetened drinks can rapidly increase blood sugar due to their high sugar content and quick absorption.

2. **Candy and Sweets:** Confections like candies, chocolates, and desserts are often loaded with refined sugars, causing a swift spike in blood glucose.

3. **Processed Snacks:** Many commercially available snacks, such as chips and cookies, contain refined carbohydrates and sugars that can lead to elevated blood sugar levels.

4. **White Bread and Pastries:** Foods made with refined white flour, such as white bread and pastries, lack fiber and can result in a rapid increase in blood sugar.

5. **Sweetened Breakfast Cereals:** Cereals with added sugars can contribute to high blood sugar levels, especially when consumed in large quantities.

6. **Flavored Yogurts:** Flavored yogurts often contain added sugars, impacting blood sugar. Opting for plain, unsweetened varieties is a healthier choice.

7. **Certain Fruits:** While fruits are generally healthy, some have higher sugar content. Limiting intake of fruits like watermelon, pineapples, and ripe bananas can help manage blood sugar.

8. **Dried Fruits:** Drying concentrates the sugars in fruits, making dried fruits like raisins and dates dense in sugar and potentially causing blood sugar spikes.

9. **Sweetened Condiments**: Condiments like ketchup, barbecue sauce, and sweet dressings can contain hidden sugars that contribute to elevated blood glucose levels.

10. **Honey and Maple Syrup:** Natural sweeteners like honey and maple syrup, while perceived as healthier alternatives, can still raise blood sugar levels significantly.

11. **Instant and Flavored Oatmeal:** Some instant oatmeal varieties and flavored oatmeal packets contain added sugars that can impact blood sugar levels.

12. **Alcohol Mixers:** Cocktails and mixed drinks often contain sugary mixers, leading to a rapid increase in blood glucose levels.

13. **Regular Pasta:** Refined pasta lacks fiber, causing a quicker spike in blood sugar. Opting for whole-grain or alternative pasta options is a better choice.

14. **Certain Sauces:** Sweetened sauces like teriyaki, hoisin, and some barbecue sauces can contribute to elevated blood sugar due to added sugars.

15. **Potato Products:** Processed potato products like fries and chips have a high glycemic index, leading to rapid increases in blood sugar levels. Opting for whole, baked potatoes is a better choice.

HEALTHY FOODS THAT DON'T RAISE YOUR BLOOD SUGAR

1. **Leafy Greens:** Vegetables like spinach, kale, and Swiss chard are low in carbohydrates and won't spike blood sugar.

2. **Broccoli:** Rich in fiber and nutrients, broccoli has a minimal impact on blood sugar levels.

3. **Avocado:** Packed with healthy fats and fiber, avocados help stabilize blood sugar.

4. **Berries:** Blueberries, strawberries, and raspberries have low sugar content and are high in antioxidants.

5. **Nuts and Seeds:** Almonds, chia seeds, and flaxseeds provide healthy fats, protein, and fiber without causing blood sugar spikes.

6. **Fatty Fish:** Salmon, mackerel, and sardines offer omega-3 fatty acids and protein, promoting stable blood sugar.

7. **Olive Oil:** A source of monounsaturated fats, olive oil can be used for cooking or as a salad dressing without affecting blood sugar significantly.

8. **Chia Seeds:** These tiny seeds are high in fiber, promoting a gradual rise in blood sugar.

9. **Garlic:** Besides adding flavor, garlic may have blood sugar-lowering properties.

10. **Non-Starchy Vegetables:** Bell peppers, cucumbers, and cauliflower are low in carbs and won't cause rapid blood sugar elevation.

11. **Greek Yogurt:** High in protein and probiotics, Greek yogurt has a minimal impact on blood sugar.

12. **Cinnamon:** Some studies suggest that cinnamon may help improve insulin sensitivity, managing blood sugar levels.

13. **Eggs:** Rich in protein and healthy fats, eggs provide a balanced option for maintaining blood sugar.

14. **Tomatoes:** With a low glycemic index, tomatoes have a mild impact on blood sugar.

15. **Quinoa:** A whole grain that contains fiber and protein, quinoa has a slower impact on blood sugar compared to refined grains.

5 KEY SUPPLEMENTS FOR A HEALTHY PREGNANCY

1. **Folic Acid (Folate):** Essential for neural tube development in early pregnancy, folic acid helps

prevent birth defects. It's crucial, especially during the first trimester.

2. **Iron:** Pregnant women often need more iron to support the increased blood volume and prevent iron-deficiency anemia. Iron supports the transport of oxygen to the developing baby.

3. **Calcium:** Vital for the development of the baby's bones, teeth, and muscles. If dietary intake is insufficient, a calcium supplement may be recommended.

4. **Omega-3 Fatty Acids:** DHA (docosahexaenoic acid) is a type of omega-3 crucial for fetal brain and eye development. It is commonly found in fish oil supplements.

5. **Vitamin D:** Important for calcium absorption and bone health, vitamin D is essential during pregnancy. It also plays a role in immune function for both the mother and baby.

SAFE EXERCISE FOR GESTATIONAL DIABETES

1. **Walking:** A low-impact exercise that helps control blood sugar levels and is suitable for various fitness levels.
2. **Swimming:** Gentle on the joints, swimming provides an effective full-body workout without excessive stress.
3. **Prenatal Yoga:** Focuses on flexibility, balance, and relaxation, promoting overall well-being during pregnancy.
4. **Pilates:** Strengthens core muscles and improves posture, aiding in the prevention of gestational diabetes complications.
5. **Stationary Cycling:** Low-impact cardiovascular exercise that helps manage blood sugar while being gentle on the joints.
6. **Prenatal Aerobics:** Tailored aerobic classes for pregnant women, promoting cardiovascular health and overall fitness.

7. **Low-Impact Aerobics:** A moderate aerobic workout that helps regulate blood sugar without high-impact stress on the body.

8. **Water Aerobics:** Combines the benefits of aerobic exercise with the buoyancy of water, reducing impact on joints.

9. **Prenatal Strength Training:** Light resistance training can help maintain muscle tone and support overall health during pregnancy.

10. **Modified Squats:** Strengthen leg and core muscles with squats, ensuring proper form and avoiding excessive strain.

11. **Pelvic Floor Exercises (Kegels):** Aid in pelvic muscle strength, which can be beneficial during pregnancy and labor.

12. **Seated Leg Lifts:** A safe way to strengthen leg muscles without putting stress on the back.

13. **Modified Planks:** Strengthening the core with modified planks can provide stability without excessive strain.

14. **Wall Push-Ups:** Offer an upper body workout without the pressure on the abdominal region.

CHAPTER 2

14-DAY MEAL PLAN

DAY 1

Breakfast: Cranberry-Almond Granola Bars

Lunch: Greek Chicken Meatballs

Dinner: Salmon Rice Bowl

DAY 2

Breakfast: Blueberry Almond Chia Pudding

Lunch: Chicken Hummus Bowl

Dinner: Spinach Salad with Warm Bacon

DAY 3

Breakfast: Veggie Omelet

Lunch: Carne Asada Burrito Bowl

Dinner: Quinoa, Avocado & Chickpea Salad over Mixed Greens

DAY 4

Breakfast: Oatmeal with Cinnamon

Lunch: Chicken Veggie Stir Fry

Dinner: Camarones a la Criolla (Shrimp in Creole Sauce)

DAY 5

Breakfast: Mango-Almond Smoothie Bowl

Lunch: Vegetarian Lentil Tacos

Dinner: Winter Greens Bowl

DAY 6

Breakfast: Breakfast Tostada

Lunch: Lemon Garlic Salmon

Dinner: Pan-Seared Steak with Crispy Herbs & Escarole

DAY 7

Breakfast: Callaloo Frittata

Lunch: Easy Quinoa Salad

Dinner: California Turkey Burgers & Baked Sweet Potato Fries

DAY 8

Breakfast: Vanilla-Cranberry Overnight Oatmeal

Lunch: Mexican Chopped Salad

Dinner: Baked Halibut with Brussels Sprouts & Quinoa

DAY 9

Breakfast: Apple Cinnamon Chia Pudding

Lunch: Veggie and Hummus Sandwich

Dinner: Grilled Eggplant & Tomato Quinoa Bowl

DAY 10

Lunch: Salmon Noodles Casserole

Dinner: Kale & Avocado Salad with Blueberries & Edamame

DAY 11

Breakfast: Cranberry-Almond Granola Bars

Lunch: Greek Chicken Meatballs

Dinner: Salmon Rice Bowl

DAY 12

Breakfast: Blueberry Almond Chia Pudding

Lunch: Chicken Hummus Bowl

Dinner: Spinach Salad with Warm Bacon

DAY 13

Breakfast: Veggie Omelet

Lunch: Carne Asada Burrito Bowl

Dinner: Quinoa, Avocado & Chickpea Salad over Mixed Greens

DAY 14

Breakfast: Oatmeal with Cinnamon

Lunch: Chicken Veggie Stir Fry

Dinner: Camarones a la Criolla (Shrimp in Creole Sauce)

CHAPTER 3

NUTRITIOUS RECIPES
GESTATIONAL DIABETES DIET

BREAKFAST

Chai Chia Pudding

Preparation Time: 10 minutes

Serves:3

Protein: 5g **Carbs:** 15g **Fiber:** 7g **Sodium:** 70mg **Calories:** 120 **Sugar:** 5g

Ingredients:

3 tablespoons chia seeds

1 cup unsweetened almond milk

1 teaspoon chai spice blend (cinnamon, cardamom, ginger, cloves)

1/4 teaspoon vanilla extract

1/4 cup chopped nuts (almonds, walnuts) for topping

Fresh berries for garnish

Method of Preparation:

1. In a bowl, mix chia seeds, almond milk, chai spice blend, and vanilla extract.
2. Stir well and let it sit for 5 minutes, then stir again to prevent clumping.
3. Refrigerate for at least 2 hours or overnight until a pudding-like consistency is achieved.
4. Before serving, top with chopped nuts and fresh berries.

Cranberry-Almond Granola Bars

Serves: 3

Preparation Time: 20 minutes

Protein: 6g **Carbs:** 30g **Fiber:** 4g **Sodium:** 50mg **Calories:** 220 **Sugar:** 12g

Ingredients:

1 cup rolled oats

1/2 cup almonds, chopped

1/4 cup dried cranberries (unsweetened)

1/4 cup almond butter

1/2 teaspoon vanilla extract

A pinch of salt

Method of Preparation:

1. Preheat oven to 350°F (175°C) and line a small baking dish with parchment paper.
2. In a bowl, combine oats, chopped almonds, and dried cranberries.
3. In a small saucepan, heat almond butter, vanilla extract, and salt over low heat until well combined.
4. Pour the wet mixture over the dry ingredients and mix until everything is evenly coated.
5. Press the mixture firmly into the prepared baking dish.
6. Bake for 15 minutes or until the edges are golden brown.

Allow to cool before cutting into bars.

Blueberry Almond Chia Pudding

Preparation Time: 15 minutes

Serves:3

Protein: 4g **Carbs:** 18g **Fiber:** 8g **Sodium:** 80mg **Calories:** 130 **Sugar:** 7g

Ingredients:

3 tablespoons chia seeds

1 cup unsweetened almond milk

1/2 cup fresh blueberries

1/4 teaspoon almond extract

Sliced almonds for topping

Method of Preparation:

1. In a bowl, combine chia seeds, almond milk, blueberries, and almond extract.

2. Stir well and let it sit for 5 minutes, then stir again to prevent clumping.

3. Refrigerate for at least 1 hour or until a pudding-like consistency is achieved.

4. Before serving, top with sliced almonds.

Veggie Omelet

Preparation Time: 15 minutes

Serves:3

Protein: 12g **Carbs:** 5g **Fiber:** 1g **Sodium:** 220mg
Calories: 160 **Sugar:** 2g

Ingredients:

3 large eggs

1/4 cup diced bell peppers (red, green, or yellow)

1/4 cup diced tomatoes

1/4 cup diced onions

1/4 cup spinach, chopped

1 tablespoon olive oil

A pinch salt and pepper

Method of Preparation:

1. In a bowl, whisk eggs and season with salt and pepper.

2. Heat olive oil in a non-stick skillet over medium heat.

3. Add diced bell peppers, tomatoes, onions, and chopped spinach to the skillet.

4. Cook until veggies are tender, about 3-4 minutes.

5. Pour the whisked eggs over the veggies, ensuring even distribution.

6. Allow the omelet to set for a minute, then gently lift the edges and tilt the pan to let the uncooked eggs flow to the edges.

7. Once the eggs are mostly set, carefully flip the omelet.

8. Cook for an additional 1-2 minutes or until the eggs are cooked through.

9. Fold the omelet in half and serve.

Oatmeal with Cinnamon

Preparation Time: 15 minutes

Serves: 3

Protein: 6g **Carbs:** 30g **Fiber:** 5g **Sodium:** 10mg **Calories:** 180 **Sugar:** 1g

Ingredients:

1 cup rolled oats

2 cups water

1/2 teaspoon ground cinnamon

1 tablespoon chia seeds

1/4 cup unsweetened almond milk

Fresh berries for topping

Method of Preparation:

1. In a saucepan, bring water to a boil, then stir in rolled oats.
2. Reduce heat to low and simmer for 5-7 minutes, stirring occasionally.
3. Add ground cinnamon and chia seeds, stirring until well combined.
4. Cook for an additional 2-3 minutes until the oats are creamy and fully cooked.
5. Remove from heat and stir in almond milk.
6. Serve hot, topped with fresh berries.

Mango-Almond Smoothie Bowl

Preparation Time: 10 minutes

Serves: 3

Protein: 8g **Carbs:** 30g **Fiber:** 5g **Sodium:** 70mg **Calories:** 210 **Sugar:** 20g

Ingredients:

1 cup frozen mango chunks

1/2 banana

1/2 cup unsweetened almond milk

1/4 cup plain Greek yogurt

1 tablespoon almond butter

Toppings: Sliced almonds, fresh mango chunks, chia seeds

Method of Preparation:

1. In a blender, combine frozen mango chunks, banana, almond milk, Greek yogurt, and almond butter.
2. Blend until smooth and creamy.
3. Pour into bowls and top with sliced almonds, fresh mango chunks, and chia seeds.

Breakfast Tostada

Preparation Time: 15 minutes

Serves:3

Protein: 10g **Carbs:** 25g **Fiber:** 7g **Sodium:** 240mg
Calories: 200 **Sugar:** 2g

Ingredients:

3 corn tostadas

3 large eggs, scrambled

1/2 cup black beans, drained and rinsed

1/4 cup diced tomatoes

1/4 cup diced avocado

1 tablespoon chopped cilantro

Salsa for topping

Method of Preparation:

1. Heat the tostadas in a dry skillet over medium heat until they are warm and slightly crispy.

2. Scramble the eggs in a separate skillet until fully cooked.

3. Assemble the tostadas by spreading black beans on each tostada, then topping with scrambled eggs,

diced tomatoes, diced avocado, and chopped cilantro.

4. Finish with a dollop of salsa on top.

Callaloo Frittata

Preparation Time: 20 minutes

Serves:3

Protein: 14g **Carbs:** 5g **Fiber:** 2g **Sodium:** 290mg **Calories:** 220 **Sugar:** 1g

Ingredients:

6 large eggs

1 cup fresh callaloo leaves, chopped

1/4 cup diced bell peppers (any color)

1/4 cup diced onions

1/4 cup shredded Parmesan cheese

1 tablespoon olive oil

Method of Preparation:

1. Preheat the oven to 375°F (190°C).

2. In an oven-safe skillet, sauté onions and bell peppers in olive oil until softened.

3. Add chopped callaloo leaves and cook until wilted.

4. In a bowl, whisk eggs, salt, and pepper. Pour the mixture over the veggies in the skillet.

5. Sprinkle shredded Parmesan cheese on top.

6. Cook on the stovetop for 2-3 minutes, then transfer to the preheated oven and bake for 10-12 minutes or until the frittata is set.

Vanilla-Cranberry Overnight Oatmeal

Preparation Time: 10 minutes

Serves:3

Protein: 6g **Carbs:** 35g **Fiber:** 7g **Sodium:** 80mg **Calories:** 220 **Sugar:** 6g

Ingredients:

1 cup rolled oats

1 cup unsweetened almond milk

1/2 cup fresh cranberries

1 teaspoon vanilla extract

Chopped nuts for topping

Method of Preparation:

1. In a bowl, mix rolled oats, almond milk, cranberries, and vanilla extract.
2. Divide the mixture into three jars or bowls and refrigerate overnight.
3. In the morning, give it a good stir and top with chopped nuts before serving.

Apple Cinnamon Chia Pudding

Preparation Time: 15 minutes

Serves:3

Protein: 5g **Carbs:** 20g **Fiber:** 8g **Sodium:** 60mg **Calories:** 150 **Sugar:** 10g

Ingredients:

3 tablespoons chia seeds

1 cup unsweetened almond milk

1/2 cup grated apple

1/2 teaspoon ground cinnamon

Sliced apples for topping

Method of Preparation:

1. In a bowl, combine chia seeds, almond milk, grated apple, and ground cinnamon.
2. Stir well and let it sit for 5 minutes, then stir again to prevent clumping.
3. Refrigerate for at least 1 hour or until a pudding-like consistency is achieved.
4. Before serving, top with sliced apples.

LUNCH

Greek Chicken Meatballs

Preparation Time: 20 minutes

Serves: 3

Protein: 25g **Carbs:** 10g **Fiber:** 1g **Sodium:** 360mg **Calories:** 280 **Sugar:** 2g

Ingredients:

1-pound ground chicken

1/4 cup breadcrumbs (use whole wheat if available)

1/4 cup crumbled feta cheese

1/4 cup finely chopped red onion

1 tablespoon fresh mint, chopped

1 tablespoon fresh parsley, chopped

1 teaspoon dried oregano

1/2 teaspoon garlic powder

A pinch salt and pepper

Tzatziki sauce for serving

Method of Preparation:

1. Preheat the oven to 400°F (200°C).
2. In a large bowl, combine ground chicken, breadcrumbs, feta cheese, red onion, mint, parsley, oregano, garlic powder, salt, and pepper.
3. Mix until well combined, then form into meatballs.
4. Place the meatballs on a baking sheet and bake for 15-18 minutes or until fully cooked.
5. Serve with tzatziki sauce on the side.

Chicken Hummus Bowl

Preparation Time: 25 minutes

Serves:3

Protein: 30g **Carbs:** 30g **Fiber:** 7g **Sodium:** 470mg
Calories: 360 **Sugar:** 3g

Ingredients:

1-pound boneless, skinless chicken breasts, grilled and sliced

1 cup cooked quinoa

1 cup cherry tomatoes, halved

1 cucumber, diced

1/4 cup Kalamata olives, sliced

1/4 cup red onion, thinly sliced

1/2 cup hummus

Fresh parsley for garnish

Method of Preparation:

1. Grill chicken breasts until fully cooked, then slice into strips.

2. Assemble the bowl by dividing quinoa, grilled chicken, cherry tomatoes, cucumber, Kalamata olives, and red onion among three bowls.

3. Top each bowl with a dollop of hummus and garnish with fresh parsley.

Carne Asada Burrito Bowl

Preparation Time: 25 minutes

Serves:3

Protein: 28g **Carbs:** 40g **Fiber:** 9g **Sodium:** 350mg **Calories:** 420 **Sugar:** 3g

Ingredients:

1-pound carne asada (grilled and sliced steak)

1 cup cooked brown rice

1 cup black beans, drained and rinsed

1 cup corn kernels (fresh or frozen)

1 cup cherry tomatoes, halved

1 avocado, sliced

Fresh cilantro for garnish

Lime wedges for serving

Method of Preparation:

1. Grill carne asada until fully cooked, then slice into strips.
2. Assemble the bowl by dividing brown rice, carne asada, black beans, corn, cherry tomatoes, and avocado among three bowls.
3. Garnish with fresh cilantro and serve with lime wedges on the side.

Chicken Veggie Stir Fry

Preparation Time: 20 minutes

Serves: 3

Protein: 25g **Carbs:** 15g **Fiber:** 4g **Sodium:** 760mg **Calories:** 300 **Sugar:** 4g

Ingredients:

1-pound boneless, skinless chicken breasts, thinly sliced

2 cups broccoli florets

1 bell pepper, thinly sliced

1 carrot, julienned

1 cup snap peas, ends trimmed

3 tablespoons low-sodium soy sauce

2 tablespoons oyster sauce

1 tablespoon sesame oil

1 tablespoon cornstarch

2 cloves garlic, minced

1 teaspoon fresh ginger, grated

2 tablespoons vegetable oil

Sesame seeds for garnish

Method of Preparation:

1. In a small bowl, whisk together soy sauce, oyster sauce, sesame oil, cornstarch, minced garlic, and grated ginger to make the sauce.

2. Heat vegetable oil in a wok or large skillet over medium-high heat.

3. Add sliced chicken and stir-fry until browned and cooked through.

4. Add broccoli, bell pepper, carrot, and snap peas to the wok. Stir-fry for 3-4 minutes until veggies are tender-crisp.

5. Pour the sauce over the chicken and veggies, stirring to coat evenly.

6. Continue to stir-fry for an additional 2-3 minutes until the sauce thickens.

7. Garnish with sesame seeds and serve.

Vegetarian Lentil Tacos

Preparation Time: 20 minutes

Serves: 3

Protein: 12g **Carbs:** 35g **Fiber:** 10g **Sodium:** 320mg **Calories:** 250 **Sugar:** 4g

Ingredients:

1 cup cooked lentils

1 tablespoon olive oil

1 small onion, diced

2 cloves garlic, minced

1 tablespoon taco seasoning

1/2 cup tomato sauce

Corn or whole wheat tortillas

Toppings: Shredded lettuce, diced tomatoes, avocado slices, cilantro

Method of Preparation:

1. Heat olive oil in a skillet over medium heat.
2. Add diced onions and garlic, sauté until softened.
3. Stir in cooked lentils and taco seasoning, mixing well.
4. Pour in tomato sauce and cook for an additional 5 minutes until heated through.
5. Warm tortillas and spoon lentil mixture onto each.
6. Top with shredded lettuce, diced tomatoes, avocado slices, and cilantro.

Lemon Garlic Salmon

Preparation Time: 20 minutes

Serves: 3

Protein: 25g **Carbs:** 1g **Fiber:** 0g **Sodium:** 150mg
Calories: 280 **Sugar:** 0g

Ingredients:

3 salmon fillets

2 tablespoons olive oil

3 cloves garlic, minced

Zest of 1 lemon

Juice of 1 lemon

1 teaspoon dried oregano

A pinch salt and pepper

Fresh parsley for garnish

Method of Preparation:

1. Preheat the oven to 400°F (200°C).

2. Place salmon fillets on a baking sheet lined with parchment paper.

3. In a small bowl, mix olive oil, minced garlic, lemon zest, lemon juice, dried oregano, salt, and pepper.

4. Brush the lemon garlic mixture over the salmon fillets.

5. Bake for 15-18 minutes or until the salmon flakes easily with a fork.

6. Garnish with fresh parsley before serving.

Easy Quinoa Salad

Preparation Time: 15 minutes

Serves:3

Protein: 7g **Carbs:** 35g **Fiber:** 5g **Sodium:** 160mg **Calories:** 260 **Sugar:** 3g

Ingredients:

1 cup quinoa, cooked and cooled

1 cup cherry tomatoes, halved

1 cucumber, diced

1/2 cup red bell pepper, diced

1/4 cup red onion, finely chopped

1/4 cup feta cheese, crumbled

2 tablespoons olive oil

1 tablespoon balsamic vinegar

A pinch salt and pepper

Fresh basil leaves for garnish

Method of Preparation:

1. In a large bowl, combine cooked quinoa, cherry tomatoes, cucumber, red bell pepper, red onion, and feta cheese.
2. In a small bowl, whisk together olive oil, balsamic vinegar, salt, and pepper.
3. Pour the dressing over the quinoa mixture and toss to combine.
4. Garnish with fresh basil leaves before serving.

Mexican Chopped Salad

Preparation Time: 15 minutes

Serves:3

Protein: 9g **Carbs:** 30g **Fiber:** 9g **Sodium:** 320mg
Calories: 270 **Sugar:** 4g

Ingredients:

4 cups mixed greens (romaine, spinach, arugula)

1 cup cherry tomatoes, halved

1 cup black beans, drained and rinsed

1 cup corn kernels (fresh or frozen)

1/2 cup red onion, finely chopped

1 avocado, diced

1/4 cup cilantro, chopped

1 lime, juiced

2 tablespoons olive oil

1 teaspoon ground cumin

A pinch salt and pepper

Tortilla strips for garnish

Method of Preparation:

1. In a large bowl, combine mixed greens, cherry tomatoes, black beans, corn, red onion, avocado, and cilantro.

2. In a small bowl, whisk together lime juice, olive oil, ground cumin, salt, and pepper.

3. Drizzle the dressing over the salad and toss to combine.

4. Garnish with tortilla strips before serving.

Veggie and Hummus Sandwich

Preparation Time: 10 minutes

Serves:3

Protein: 10g **Carbs:** 45g **Fiber:** 9g **Sodium:** 550mg **Calories:** 320 **Sugar:** 7g

Ingredients:

6 slices whole grain bread

1 cup hummus

1 cucumber, thinly sliced

1 tomato, thinly sliced

1/2 red bell pepper, thinly sliced

1/4 red onion, thinly sliced

1 cup mixed greens (spinach, arugula)

A pinch salt and pepper

Method of Preparation:

1. Spread hummus evenly on each slice of bread.
2. Layer cucumber, tomato, red bell pepper, red onion, and mixed greens on half of the bread slices.
3. Sprinkle with A pinch salt and pepper.
4. Top with the remaining bread slices to make sandwiches.

Salmon Noodles Casserole

Preparation Time: 25 minutes

Serves:3

Protein: 30g **Carbs:** 40g **Fiber:** 8g **Sodium:** 320mg **Calories:** 420 **Sugar:** 4g

Ingredients:

8 oz whole wheat noodles, cooked

3 salmon fillets, cooked and flaked

1 cup broccoli florets, steamed

1 cup cherry tomatoes, halved

1/2 cup plain Greek yogurt

1/4 cup grated Parmesan cheese

2 tablespoons whole wheat flour

2 tablespoons olive oil

2 cloves garlic, minced

1 teaspoon lemon zest

A pinch salt and pepper

Method of Preparation:

1. Preheat the oven to 375°F (190°C).
2. In a large bowl, combine cooked noodles, flaked salmon, steamed broccoli, and cherry tomatoes.
3. In a saucepan, heat olive oil and sauté minced garlic until fragrant.
4. Stir in whole wheat flour, then gradually whisk in Greek yogurt until smooth.
5. Add Parmesan cheese, lemon zest, salt, and pepper. Cook until the sauce thickens.
6. Pour the sauce over the noodle mixture and toss to coat evenly.

7. Transfer to a baking dish and bake for 15-20 minutes or until the top is golden brown.

Dinner

Kale & Avocado Salad with Blueberries & Edamame

Preparation Time: 15 minutes

Serves:3

Protein: 9g **Carbs:** 20g **Fiber:** 8g **Sodium:** 160mg **Calories:** 280 **Sugar:** 8g

Ingredients:

4 cups kale, stems removed and chopped

1 avocado, diced

1 cup blueberries

1/2 cup edamame, cooked and shelled

1/4 cup feta cheese, crumbled

2 tablespoons olive oil

1 tablespoon balsamic vinegar

A pinch salt and pepper

Method of Preparation:

1. In a large bowl, combine kale, diced avocado, blueberries, edamame, and crumbled feta cheese.
2. In a small bowl, whisk together olive oil, balsamic vinegar, salt, and pepper.
3. Pour the dressing over the salad and toss to coat.

Salmon Cauliflower Rice Bowl

Preparation Time: 25 minutes

Serves:3

Protein: 30g **Carbs:** 40g **Fiber:** 8g **Sodium:** 600mg **Calories:** 420 **Sugar:** 3g

Ingredients:

3 salmon fillets, grilled or baked

2 cups cooked Cauliflower rice

1 cup broccoli florets, steamed

1 carrot, julienned

1/2 cucumber, thinly sliced

1 avocado, sliced

2 tablespoons soy sauce

1 tablespoon sesame oil

1 tablespoon rice vinegar

Sesame seeds for garnish

Green onions for garnish

Method of Preparation:

1. Grill or bake salmon fillets until fully cooked.
2. In a bowl, assemble cooked cauliflower rice, steamed broccoli, julienned carrot, sliced cucumber, and avocado.
3. In a small bowl, whisk together soy sauce, sesame oil, and rice vinegar.
4. Drizzle the sauce over the rice bowl.
5. Top with grilled or baked salmon fillets.
6. Garnish with sesame seeds and green onions.

Spinach Salad with Warm Bacon

Preparation Time: 15 minutes

Serves: 3

Protein: 8g **Carbs:** 10g **Fiber:** 4g **Sodium:** 420mg
Calories: 200 **Sugar:** 2g

Ingredients:

6 cups fresh spinach

4 slices bacon, cooked and crumbled

1 cup cherry tomatoes, halved

1/4 cup red onion, thinly sliced

1/4 cup feta cheese, crumbled

2 tablespoons olive oil

1 tablespoon red wine vinegar

1 teaspoon Dijon mustard

A pinch salt and pepper

Method of Preparation:

1. In a large salad bowl, combine fresh spinach, crumbled bacon, cherry tomatoes, red onion, and crumbled feta cheese.

2. In a small bowl, whisk together olive oil, red wine vinegar, Dijon mustard, salt, and pepper.

3. Drizzle the dressing over the salad and toss to coat.

4. Serve immediately, and enjoy the warm bacon flavor.

Quinoa, Avocado & Chickpea Salad over Mixed Greens

Preparation Time: 20 minutes

Serves:3

Protein: 10g **Carbs:** 40g **Fiber:** 10g **Sodium:** 280mg **Calories:** 340g **Sugar:** 3g

Ingredients:

1 cup quinoa, cooked and cooled

1 avocado, diced

1 can (15 oz) chickpeas, drained and rinsed

4 cups mixed greens (arugula, spinach, kale)

1/4 cup red onion, finely chopped

1/4 cup fresh cilantro, chopped

2 tablespoons olive oil

1 tablespoon lime juice

1 teaspoon cumin

A pinch salt and pepper

Method of Preparation:

1. In a large bowl, combine quinoa, diced avocado, chickpeas, mixed greens, red onion, and cilantro.
2. In a small bowl, whisk together olive oil, lime juice, cumin, salt, and pepper.
3. Drizzle the dressing over the salad and toss gently to combine.

Camarones a la Criolla (Shrimp in Creole Sauce)

Preparation Time: 25 minutes

Serves:3

Protein: 20g **Carbs:** 15g **Fiber:** 3g **Sodium:** 580mg **Calories:** 230 **Sugar:** 6g

Ingredients:

1-pound large shrimp, peeled and deveined

1 tablespoon olive oil

1 onion, finely chopped

1 bell pepper, diced

2 cloves garlic, minced

1 can (14 oz) diced tomatoes

1/4 cup tomato sauce

1 teaspoon dried oregano

1 teaspoon paprika

1/2 teaspoon cayenne pepper (adjust to taste)

A pinch salt and pepper

Fresh cilantro for garnish

Cooked brown rice for serving

Method of Preparation:

1. In a large skillet, heat olive oil over medium heat.
2. Sauté chopped onion and bell pepper until softened.
3. Add minced garlic and cook for an additional minute.

4. Stir in diced tomatoes, tomato sauce, oregano, paprika, cayenne pepper, salt, and pepper.

5. Simmer for 10-12 minutes until the sauce thickens.

6. Add peeled and deveined shrimp, cooking for 5-7 minutes until the shrimp are pink and fully cooked.

7. Serve over cooked brown rice and garnish with fresh cilantro.

Winter Greens Bowl

Preparation Time: 25 minutes

Serves: 3

Protein: 5g **Carbs:** 30g **Fiber:** 8g **Sodium:** 150mg **Calories:** 280 **Sugar:** 10g

Ingredients:

4 cups winter greens (kale, Swiss chard, collard greens), chopped

1 cup butternut squash, diced and roasted

1 cup Brussels sprouts, halved and roasted

1/4 cup pomegranate seeds

1/4 cup pecans, toasted and chopped

2 tablespoons olive oil

1 tablespoon balsamic vinegar

Method of Preparation:

1. In a large bowl, combine chopped winter greens, diced and roasted butternut squash, roasted Brussels sprouts, pomegranate seeds, and toasted pecans.
2. In a small bowl, whisk together olive oil, balsamic vinegar, salt, and pepper.
3. Drizzle the dressing over the greens bowl and toss gently to combine.

Pan-Seared Steak with Crispy Herbs & Escarole

Preparation Time: 25 minutes

Serves: 3

Protein: 35g **Carbs:** 2g **Fiber:** 1g **Sodium:** 100mg **Calories:** 320 **Sugar:** 1g

Ingredients:

3 sirloin steaks

2 tablespoons olive oil

3 cloves garlic, minced

2 tablespoons fresh rosemary, chopped

2 tablespoons fresh thyme, chopped

A pinch salt and pepper

1 head escarole, washed and chopped

Method of Preparation:

1. Pat the steaks dry and season with salt and pepper.
2. In a large skillet, heat olive oil over medium-high heat.
3. Sear the steak for 3-4 minutes per side for medium-rare, or adjust to your liking.
4. In the last minute of cooking, add minced garlic, rosemary, and thyme to the pan, allowing the herbs to crisp up.
5. Remove the steaks and let them rest.
6. In the same skillet, add chopped escarole and sauté until wilted.

7. Serve the steaks over a bed of crispy herbs and escarole.

California Turkey Burgers & Baked Potato Fries

Preparation Time: 30 minutes

Serves:3

Protein: 25g   **Carbs:** 30g **Fiber:**   5g **Sodium:** 320mg **Calories:** 330g **Sugar:** 4g

Ingredients:

For Turkey Burgers:

1-pound ground turkey

1/4 cup breadcrumbs (use whole wheat if available)

1/4 cup red onion, finely chopped

1/4 cup cilantro, chopped

1 teaspoon cumin

For Baked Sweet Potato Fries:

2 large potatoes, cut into fries

2 tablespoons olive oil

1 teaspoon smoked paprika

Method of Preparation:

1. Preheat the oven to 400°F (200°C).
2. In a bowl, mix ground turkey, breadcrumbs, red onion, cilantro, cumin, salt, and pepper.
3. Form into patties.
4. Grill or cook turkey burgers on a stovetop until fully cooked.
5. Toss potato fries with olive oil, smoked paprika, and salt.
6. Arrange on a baking sheet.
7. Bake sweet potato fries for 20-25 minutes or until crispy.

Baked Halibut with Brussels Sprouts & Quinoa

Preparation Time: 30 minutes

Serves: 3

Protein: 30g **Carbs:** 35g **Fiber:** 8g **Sodium:** 200mg **Calories:** 350 **Sugar:** 6g

Ingredients:

3 halibut fillets

1-pound Brussels sprouts, trimmed and halved

1 cup quinoa, cooked

2 tablespoons olive oil

1 tablespoon Dijon mustard

1 teaspoon lemon zest

A pinch salt and pepper

Method of Preparation:

1. Preheat the oven to 375°F (190°C).
2. Season halibut fillets with salt and pepper and place on a baking sheet.
3. Toss Brussels sprouts with olive oil, salt, and pepper. Arrange around the halibut.
4. In a small bowl, whisk together Dijon mustard, and lemon zest. Brush over the halibut fillets.

5. Bake for 20-25 minutes or until the fish is cooked through and the Brussels sprouts are tender.

Grilled Eggplant & Tomato Quinoa Bowl

Preparation Time: 25 minutes

Serves:3

Protein: 8g **Carbs:** 35g **Fiber:** 6g **Sodium:** 240mg **Calories:** 290 **Sugar:** 4g

Ingredients:

1 large eggplant, sliced

2 tomatoes, sliced

1 cup quinoa, cooked

1/4 cup feta cheese, crumbled

2 tablespoons balsamic vinegar

2 tablespoons olive oil

1 teaspoon dried oregano

A pinch salt and pepper

Instant Pot Chicken Burrito Bowl

Preparation Time: 25 minutes

Serves:3

Protein: 30g **Carbs:** 45g **Fiber:** 9g **Sodium:** 750mg
Calories: 400 **Sugar:** 4g

Ingredients:

1-pound boneless, skinless chicken breasts, diced

1 cup brown rice, uncooked

1 can (15 oz) black beans, drained and rinsed

1 cup corn kernels (fresh or frozen)

1 cup salsa

1 cup chicken broth

1 teaspoon cumin

1 teaspoon chili powder

1 teaspoon garlic powder

A pinch salt and pepper

Toppings: Avocado, shredded cheese, cilantro, lime wedges

Method of Preparation:

1. In the Instant Pot, combine diced chicken, brown rice, black beans, corn, salsa, chicken broth, cumin, chili powder, garlic powder, salt, and pepper.
2. Seal the Instant Pot and set it to cook on high pressure for 12 minutes.
3. Allow for a natural release for 5 minutes, then release any remaining pressure manually.
4. Stir the mixture and serve in bowls.
5. Top with avocado, shredded cheese, cilantro, and a squeeze of lime.

Baked Parmesan Chicken

Preparation Time: 30 minutes

Serves:3

Protein: 30g **Carbs:** 15g **Fiber:** 2g **Sodium:** 500mg
Calories: 320 **Sugar:** 1g

Ingredients:

3 boneless, skinless chicken breasts

1 cup breadcrumbs (use whole wheat if available)

1/2 cup grated Parmesan cheese

1 teaspoon dried oregano

1 teaspoon garlic powder

A pinch salt and pepper

2 eggs, beaten

Olive oil spray

Method of Preparation:

1. Preheat the oven to 400°F (200°C) and line a baking sheet with parchment paper.
2. In a shallow bowl, mix breadcrumbs, grated Parmesan cheese, dried oregano, garlic powder, salt, and pepper.
3. Dip each chicken breast into beaten eggs, then coat with the breadcrumb mixture.
4. Place the coated chicken breasts on the prepared baking sheet.

5. Lightly spray the chicken with olive oil.

6. Bake for 20-25 minutes or until the chicken is cooked through and golden brown.

Chicken Noodles

Preparation Time: 20 minutes

Serves:3

Protein: 20g **Carbs:** 35g **Fiber:** 4g **Sodium:** 650mg
Calories: 380g **Sugar:** 3g

Ingredients:

8 oz egg noodles

1-pound boneless, skinless chicken thighs, thinly sliced

2 tablespoons soy sauce

1 tablespoon oyster sauce

1 tablespoon hoisin sauce

1 tablespoon sesame oil

1 tablespoon vegetable oil

2 cloves garlic, minced

1 teaspoon fresh ginger, grated

1 cup broccoli florets

1 carrot, julienned

Green onions for garnish

Method of Preparation:

1. Cook egg noodles according to package instructions, then drain and set aside.

2. In a bowl, mix soy sauce, oyster sauce, hoisin sauce, and sesame oil.

3. Heat vegetable oil in a wok or large skillet over medium-high heat.

4. Add minced garlic and grated ginger, sauté for 1 minute.

5. Add sliced chicken to the wok and cook until browned.

6. Add broccoli and julienned carrots, stirring until vegetables are tender-crisp.

7. Pour the sauce over the chicken and vegetables, then add the cooked noodles. Toss until everything is well-coated.

8. Garnish with green onions before serving

Turkey and Vegetable Soup

Preparation Time: 30 minutes

Serves:3

Protein: 25g **Carbs:** 15g **Fiber:** 4g **Sodium:** 600mg
Calories: 280 **Sugar:** 6g

Ingredients:

1-pound ground turkey

1 tablespoon olive oil

1 onion, diced

2 carrots, sliced

2 celery stalks, chopped

3 cloves garlic, minced

6 cups low-sodium chicken broth

1 can (14 oz) diced tomatoes, undrained

1 cup green beans, trimmed and chopped

1 cup corn kernels (fresh or frozen)

1 teaspoon dried thyme

1 teaspoon dried rosemary

A pinch salt and pepper

2 cups spinach, chopped

Method of Preparation:

1. In a large pot, cook ground turkey over medium heat until browned. Remove excess fat.
2. Add olive oil, diced onion, sliced carrots, chopped celery, and minced garlic. Sauté until vegetables are softened.
3. Pour in chicken broth, diced tomatoes, green beans, corn, dried thyme, dried rosemary, salt, and pepper.
4. Bring the soup to a boil, then reduce heat and let it simmer for 20 minutes.
5. Stir in chopped spinach and cook for an additional 5 minutes until wilted.
6. Adjust seasoning if needed and serve hot.

Oven-Fried Parmesan Chicken Drumsticks

Preparation Time: 35 minutes

Serves:3

Protein: 30g **Carbs:** 15g **Fiber:** 2g **Sodium:** 500mg **Calories:** 320 **Sugar:** 1g

Ingredients:

2 pounds chicken drumsticks

1 cup breadcrumbs (use whole wheat if available)

1/2 cup grated Parmesan cheese

1 teaspoon dried oregano

1 teaspoon garlic powder

A pinch salt and pepper

2 eggs, beaten

Olive oil spray

Method of Preparation:

1. Preheat the oven to 400°F (200°C) and line a baking sheet with parchment paper.
2. In a shallow bowl, mix breadcrumbs, grated Parmesan cheese, dried oregano, garlic powder, salt, and pepper.
3. Dip each chicken drumstick into beaten eggs, then coat with the breadcrumb mixture.
4. Place the coated drumsticks on the prepared baking sheet.
5. Lightly spray the drumsticks with olive oil.
6. Bake for 30-35 minutes or until the chicken is cooked through and the coating is crispy. Rotate the drumsticks halfway through for even cooking.

SEAFOOD MAINS

Seasoned Cod

Preparation Time: 20 minutes

Serves:3

Protein: 25g **Carbs:** 1g **Fiber:** 0g **Sodium:** 400mg
Calories: 150 **Sugar:** 0g

Ingredients:

3 cod fillets

2 tablespoons olive oil

1 teaspoon paprika

1 teaspoon garlic powder

1/2 teaspoon onion powder

1/2 teaspoon dried thyme

1/2 teaspoon dried oregano

A pinch salt and pepper

Fresh lemon wedges for serving

Method of Preparation:

1. Preheat the oven to 400°F (200°C).
2. Pat the cod fillets dry and place them on a baking sheet.
3. In a small bowl, mix olive oil, paprika, garlic powder, onion powder, dried thyme, dried oregano, salt, and pepper.

4. Brush the cod fillets with the seasoned olive oil mixture.

5. Bake for 15-18 minutes or until the cod flakes easily with a fork.

6. Serve with fresh lemon wedges.

Garlic Salmon Bites

Preparation Time: 20 minutes

Serves:3

Protein: 25g **Carbs:** 2g **Fiber:** 0g **Sodium:** 300mg **Calories:** 180 **Sugar:** 0g

Ingredients:

1-pound salmon fillet, skin removed, diced into bite-sized pieces

2 tablespoons olive oil

4 cloves garlic, minced

1 teaspoon smoked paprika

1/2 teaspoon cayenne pepper (adjust to taste)

A pinch salt and pepper

Fresh parsley for garnish

Method of Preparation:

1. In a large skillet, heat olive oil over medium heat.

2. Add minced garlic and sauté for 1-2 minutes until fragrant.

3. Add diced salmon to the skillet.

4. Season with smoked paprika, cayenne pepper, salt, and pepper.

5. Cook for 5-7 minutes, stirring gently, until salmon is cooked through.

6. Garnish with fresh parsley before serving.

Roasted Salmon with Smoky Chickpeas and Greens

Preparation Time: 25 minutes

Serves:3

Protein: 30g **Carbs:** 15g **Fiber:** 5g **Sodium:** 400mg
Calories: 280g **Sugar:** 1g

Ingredients:

3 salmon fillets

1 can (15 oz) chickpeas, drained and rinsed

2 tablespoons olive oil

1 teaspoon smoked paprika

1/2 teaspoon cumin

1/2 teaspoon garlic powder

A pinch salt and pepper

4 cups mixed greens (kale, spinach, arugula)

Lemon wedges for serving

Method of Preparation:

1. Preheat the oven to 400°F (200°C).
2. In a bowl, toss chickpeas with olive oil, smoked paprika, cumin, garlic powder, salt, and pepper.
3. Spread the chickpeas on a baking sheet.
4. Place salmon fillets on the same baking sheet.
5. Roast in the oven for 15-18 minutes or until salmon is cooked through and chickpeas are crispy.
6. Serve salmon over a bed of mixed greens, and squeeze lemon wedges over the top before serving.

Grilled Fish with Garlic Marinade

Preparation Time: 20 minutes

Serves:3

Protein: 25g **Carbs:** 2g **Fiber:** 0g **Sodium:** 300mg
Calories: 200 **Sugar:** 0g

Ingredients:

3 white fish fillets (tilapia or cod)

3 tablespoons olive oil

4 cloves garlic, minced

1 teaspoon paprika

1 teaspoon cumin

1/2 teaspoon dried oregano

A pinch salt and pepper

Fresh cilantro for garnish

Lemon wedges for serving

Method of Preparation:

1. In a small bowl, mix olive oil, minced garlic, paprika, cumin, dried oregano, salt, and pepper to create the marinade.

2. Pat the fish fillets dry and brush both sides with the marinade.

3. Let the fish marinate for at least 10 minutes.

4. Preheat the grill to medium-high heat.

5. Grill the fish for 3-4 minutes per side or until it flakes easily with a fork.

6. Garnish with fresh cilantro and serve with lemon wedges.

Cilantro Lime Shrimp Bowl

Preparation Time: 25 minutes

Serves:3

Protein: 25g **Carbs:** 45g **Fiber:** 5g **Sodium:** 300mg **Calories:** 350g **Sugar:** 1g

Ingredients:

1-pound large shrimp, peeled and deveined

2 tablespoons olive oil

Zest and juice of 2 limes

1/4 cup fresh cilantro, chopped

2 cloves garlic, minced

1 teaspoon cumin

1/2 teaspoon chili powder

A pinch salt and pepper

4 cups cooked brown rice

Avocado slices for serving

Lime wedges for serving

Method of Preparation:

1. In a bowl, combine shrimp with olive oil, lime zest, lime juice, chopped cilantro, minced garlic, cumin, chili powder, salt, and pepper. Let it marinate for 10 minutes.
2. Heat a skillet over medium-high heat.
3. Add the marinated shrimp and cook for 2-3 minutes per side or until they turn pink and opaque.

4. Serve the shrimp over cooked brown rice.

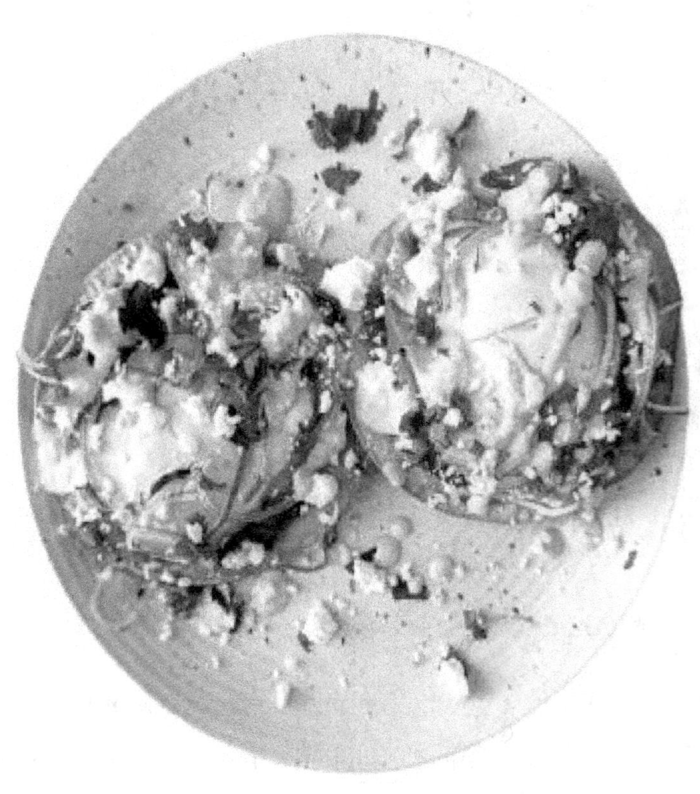

CONCLUSION

In conclusion, this cookbook serves not only as a culinary guide but as a tool for expectant mothers navigating the challenges of managing their health during pregnancy.

The recipes in this book are carefully crafted to provide delightful and nutritious options, ensuring that the journey through gestational diabetes is met with flavorful satisfaction.

Through the diverse array of recipes, this book aimed to dispel the notion that a gestational diabetes-friendly diet is synonymous with deprivation.

Instead, this cookbook encourages a celebration of wholesome ingredients, thoughtfully combined to create meals that nourish both the body and the spirit.

By emphasizing balance, portion control, and mindful food choices, it empowers mothers-to-be to savor the joy of eating while maintaining optimal blood sugar levels.

As your culinary journey concludes, it is essential to underscore the role of this cookbook in fostering a positive relationship between mothers and their nutritional choices.

Each recipe is a testament to the belief that managing gestational diabetes need not be a sacrifice but rather an opportunity to explore the rich tapestry of flavors inherent in a health-conscious lifestyle.

Furthermore, the included nutritional insights and practical tips are designed to equip you with the knowledge needed to make informed decisions about your diet beyond the confines of these pages.

The emphasis on whole foods, lean proteins, and fiber-rich ingredients ensures a well-rounded approach to nutrition, not only during pregnancy but as a foundation for a lifetime of well-being.

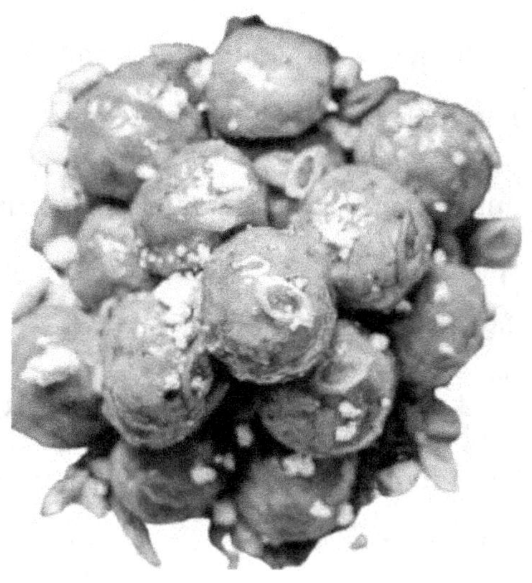